YOUR KNOWLEDGE HAS VALUE

AF149492

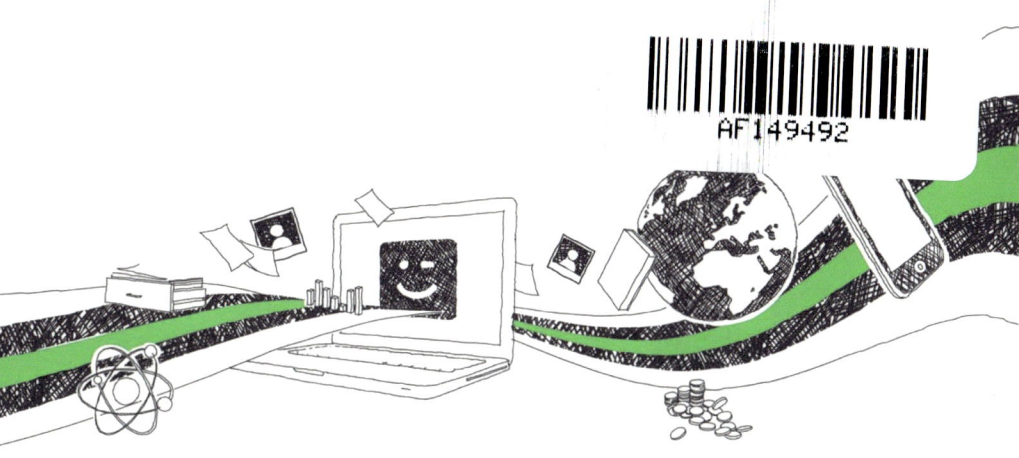

- We will publish your bachelor's and master's thesis, essays and papers

- Your own eBook and book - sold worldwide in all relevant shops

- Earn money with each sale

Upload your text at www.GRIN.com
and publish for free

Kelly Clarkson

Modeling Avian Influenza H5N1

GRIN Verlag

Bibliografische Information der Deutschen Nationalbibliothek:

Die Deutsche Bibliothek verzeichnet diese Publikation in der Deutschen National-
bibliografie; detaillierte bibliografische Daten sind im Internet über http://dnb.d-
nb.de/ abrufbar.

Imprint:

Copyright © 2012 GRIN Verlag GmbH
Druck und Bindung: Books on Demand GmbH, Norderstedt Germany
ISBN: 978-3-656-41464-3

This book at GRIN:

http://www.grin.com/en/e-book/213224/modeling-avian-influenza-h5n1

Modeling Avian Influenza H5N1

Improve SIR-Model with Virus H5N1

Introduction – Avian Influenza and Model Problem

In the recent past, bird flu has claimed many lives. These are mainly of those, belonging to humans and animals of whose food chain, birds and fowls tend to be a part. This, has in turn affected other animals, as well as upset the entire food chain. The virus has an RNA based protein (Tiensin, Thanawat, 2011), which is the cause of the problem. There are many subtypes of the virus, however only four of them have been found to be the real cause of the problems. These strains are named as the H5N1, H7N3, H7N7 and H9N2. This virus has genes, which are more adaptive towards aerial beings such as birds. However, this does not mean that the virus cannot pass on the pathogen to other beings but are relieve less likely to result in death. The World Health Organization mentions in its report that, there have been just two deaths due to Avian Flu in the countries of Egypt and Indonesia in a time span of 5th November 2012 and 17th November, 2012(World Health Organization, 2012). Both the deaths have been attributed to exposure to chicken or ducks in the backyard or in the neighborhood. In this report, we attempt to find an appropriate model so that the problem can be nipped in the bud. The report, will seek to determine the implementation and the results of various implementations in order to perfect the model. Apart from the cases reported, the avian flu has seriously hit the poultry market, with government taking no chances and introducing bans on the import and export of chicken and fowl as well as products made out of them. All the infected birds have been tested in order to eliminate chances of wrong deaths. The affected ones are out to death including their young ones and the unhatched eggs. In the fig 1.1, the table mentions the cumulative number of cases as well as deaths attributed to Avian Influenza. The table mentions data collected since 2003, the year when the flu virus first made an appearance till 2012, in order to show case the necessity for the generation of the perfect model.

Country	2003 cases	2003 deaths	2004 cases	2004 deaths	2005 cases	2005 deaths	2006 cases	2006 deaths	2007 cases	2007 deaths	2008 cases	2008 deaths	2009 cases	2009 deaths	2010 cases	2010 deaths	2011 cases	2011 deaths	2012 cases	2012 deaths	Total cases	Total deaths
Azerbaijan							8	5													8	5
Bangladesh											1						2		3		6	
Cambodia					4	4	2	2	1	1	1		1		1	1	8	8	3	3	21	19
China	1	1			8	5	13	8	5	3	4	4	7	4	2	1	1	1	2	1	43	28
Djibouti							1														1	
Egypt							18	10	25	9	8	4	39	4	29	13	39	15	11	5	169	60
Indonesia					20	13	55	45	42	37	24	20	21	19	9	7	12	10	9	9	192	160
Iraq							3	2													3	2
Lao People's Democratic Republic									2	2											2	2
Myanmar									1												1	
Nigeria									1	1											1	1
Pakistan									3	1											3	1
Thailand			17	12	5	2	3	3													25	17
Turkey							12	4													12	4
Viet Nam	3	3	29	20	61	19			8	5	6	5	5	5	7	2			4	2	123	61
Total	4	4	46	32	98	43	115	79	88	59	44	33	73	32	48	24	62	34	32	20	610	360

Total number of cases includes number of deaths WHO reports only laboratory cases
All dates refer to onset of illness

Fig 1.1 Cumulative number of confirmed human cases for avian influenza A(H5N1) reported to WHO, 2003-2012

The reasons for suggesting a mathematical model in the case of Avian Flu are listed below

- Determination of vaccines and its effectiveness can be predicted.

- The model will help us to understand the development of the virus strains and the lifecycle of the pathogens

- Such models are used for the control and the prevention of infectious disease such as Avian Flu or Swine Flu (Haran, 2009).

The mathematical model for Avian Flu is directed to understand the lifecycle of the pathogen and to aid resistant strains in order to cure the disease.

Interventions

For the control of Avian Flu there are three kinds of interventions planned which are clinical isolation of the susceptible group on people, the vaccination of the group in order to prevent the disease and administration of Tamiflu. It is important to note that the best possible intervention would be to make sure that the susceptible fowls are clinically tested (faecal matter once in every ten days to determine their condition) and isolated to prevent them from infection (Guan et all, 2007). There can be other forms of interventions as well, such as cooking poultry and fowl at the highest temperature possible in order to make sure, that the pathogen of virus strains are rendered ineffective. Other measures would be to stay away and avoid contact with domestic or wild birds of any sort and abstinence from related products (Lucchetti,Joseph; Roy, Manojit; Martcheva, Maia . 2008). Transportation of sick birds or contaminated eggs are also a way of being in contact with the disease and thus raising the susceptibility to get affected with the virus (Bhatla, Rajesh; Narain, Jai P, 2006).

Social Isolation:

One of the most tried and trusted methods of intervention, social isolation involves the limiting of social interactions on a significant scale and limits family members within their own domiciles for the duration of the infection period. Isolation also extends to limiting public gatherings, reducing the quantum of social interactions and the enforcement and facilitation of quarantines.

Social Isolation is doubly effective when implemented at the earliest stages of detection. The proper implementation of this step can significantly impede the spread of disease and limits infection and transmission to an exponential degree. According to studies, even as little as 50 percent implementation of this kind of intervention can help significantly alter patterns of influenza infection and transmission (Riley, Steven; Leung, Gabriel; Wu, Joseph)

Dynamic Vaccination

Dynamic vaccination in the case of avian flu is limited only to affected birds, the cases of bird to human transmission are so rare that they do not merit the case for serious medical research, However recently there have been developments towards formulating a human vaccine for avian flu and has recently been approved by the US food and drug administration. The fact still remains that even after such a step the amount of vaccine available does not make it a popular and widely available method for treating bird flu. Up until now vaccination still remains a secondary measure for preventing infection among humans and a primary method of stopping the infection amongst birds for which isolation is not a viable or feasible option.

Tamiflu

Tamiflu remains the WHO approved method for combating the spread of influenza. The scientific name for this drug is Oseltamivir. Oseltamivir suppresses and decreases the spread of influenza A and B viruses, the viruses responsible for the flu. It does this by blocking the action of neuraminidase, an enzyme produced by the viruses that enables the viruses to spread from infected cells to healthy cells. By preventing the spread of virus from cell to cell, the symptoms and duration of influenza infection are reduced. On average, Oseltamivir reduces the duration of symptoms by one and a half days if treatment is started within forty-eight hours of the beginning of symptoms.

Mathematical Formulation:

The SIR epidemic model is a special case of the Kernack-McKendrick model. The population is divided into three segments:

Susceptible ($S(t)$)

Infected ($I(t)$)

Removed ($R(t)$)

Susceptible individuals are those which may move on to the infected stage and after recovery may enter the removed stage, once an individual has entered the removed stage it is immune to further infection and is removed from the equation. Thus the total population may be denoted as:

$$N(t) = S(t) + I(t) + R(t)$$

The SIR model can also be expressed as a set of differential equations which are given below:

$$dS/dt = -\beta SI$$

$$dI/dt = \beta SI - \gamma I$$

$$dR/dt = \gamma I$$

However in certain cases the timescale of the epidemic outbreak is much more rapid and widespread whereas the time scale of human population is much slower, in this case the differential equation for the SIR endemic model is given in the below figure:

$$dS/dT = \Delta - \mu S - \beta S\, I/N \quad (1.1)$$

$$dI/dt = \beta S\, I/N - (\mu + _\gamma)I \quad (1.2)$$

$$dR/dt = \gamma I - \mu R \quad\quad\quad (1.3)$$

The SIR Model

Speaking of the SIR Model (Susceptible Infected Removed Model), this is one of the most popular of mathematical models, which is used for epidemics (Newman, 2002). In this model, we have three types of people namely

S_t = the number of susceptible persons in the population at time t.

I_t = the number of infected persons in the population at time t.

R_t = the number of recovered persons in the population at time t.

N = the size of the population

Another set of persons who will be a fraction of the entire population considered can be denoted in the following way

st = St÷N (the susceptible fraction of the population at time t.)

it = It÷N (the infected fraction of the population at time t.)

rt = Rt÷N (the recovered fraction of the population at time t.)

In order to understand the whole model in a better fashion, you need to keep in mind that St + It + Rt = N as well as st + it + rt = 1(since st, it and rt are fractions, therefore they should add up to 1) (Troy, 2005). Here, we present a pictorial representation of the SIR model for better comprehension wherein the letters S, I and R stand for the meaning stated above (Haran, 2009)

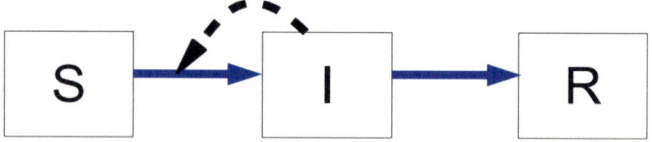

The solid arrows denote the progression of one kind of population fraction from one phase to another and the dotted arrows denotes the rate at which the susceptible class of individuals make to the category of infected beings.

Differential Equation System SIR-Model with H5N1 virus

Most of the death from Avian Influenza in humans was, when the disease was in its final stages in terms of progression. Hence, the rate of reproduction is necessary to find out in order to administer the necessary effective medicines or the intervention. There are four major mathematical model to determine the rate of reproduction which will also be helpful in determining the number of secondary cases. These models are determination by intrinsic growth rate, simple susceptible–exposed–infectious–removed model, complex susceptible–exposed–infectious–removed model and the Bayesian inference of stochastic SIR (Chowell, Gerardo; Nishiura, Hiroshi; Bettencourt,M. A., 2007).

The SIR model for Avian Influenza is not fit for those diseases in which the recovered entity can become infected again (Hethcote, 1973). Hence in this case, Rt which is the number of recovered persons in the population at time t is not considered. The equation now becomes

St + It = N

Effects of Interventions

The following graph and data is from a collection of worldwide sources and is an extrapolation of the effects of various different kinds of treatments that are employed to combat the spread of Influenza.

	Social Isolation	Dynamic Vaccination	Tamiflu	No Intervention
Early Administration	35%	5%	70%	4%
Late Administration	10%	65%	25%	0%

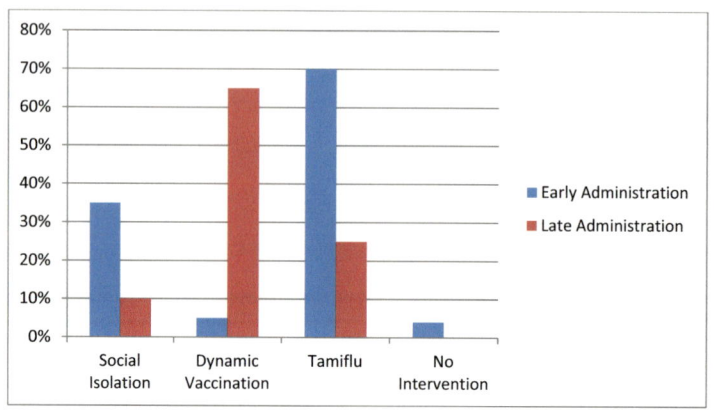

Combined interventions:

	Vaccinate 10% and isolation	Vaccinate 10% and Tamiflu	Isolation and tamiflu	All three
Adults	25%	30%	30%	15%
Children	35%	15%	20%	30%

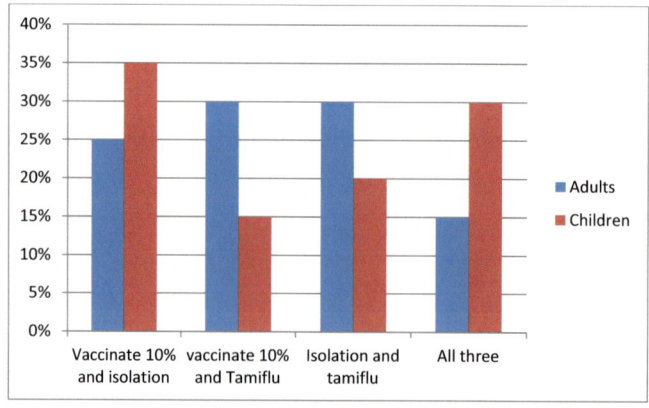

Conclusion

Avian Influenza is a disease, which primarily affects the birds and fowl. However, the strains of the pathogen are also known to have affected the human when they are exposed to the infected birds, wild or domesticated. However, the report presents a mathematical model to understand the amount of progression from one category to another, it is imperative to note that all the three interventions in conjunction can produce the desired effect. Rendering of one intervention is not possible as people in the real world may be with varying degrees of infection or are completely safe.

References

1. Bhatla, Rajesh; Narain, Jai P. (2006). Preventing Avian Influenza In Humans: The Role Of Simple Public Health Interventions . Department of Communicable Diseases. 37 (6), p1229-1236.

2. Chowell, Gerardo; Nishiura, Hiroshi; Bettencourt,M. A. (2007). Comparative estimation of the reproduction number for pandemic influenza from daily case notification data. Journal of the Royal Society Interface. 4 (12), p155-166.

3. Guan et all. (2007). BMC Infectious Diseases. Bio Med Central. - (-), -. Available at - http://www.biomedcentral.com/1471-2334/7/132

4. Hethcote, Herbert W. (1973). Asymptomic Behavior in a Deterministic Epidemic Model. Bulletin of Mathematical Biology. 35 (-), p607-614

5. Haran, Murli. (2009). An introduction to models for disease dynamics. Spatial Epidemiology SAMSI. - (-), Available at - www.unc.edu/~rls/s940/samsidisdyntut.pdf.

6. Lucchetti,Joseph; Roy, Manojit; Martcheva, Maia . (2008). An Avian Influenza Model And Its Fit To Human Avian Influenza Cases. Available: http://www.math.ufl.edu/~maia/AI_book_chapter9.pdf. Last accessed 4th Jan 2013.

7. Newman,M. E. J.. (2002). The spread of epidemic disease on networks. Center for the Study of Complex Systems. - (-), p1-11.

8. Tassier, Troy. (2005). SIR Model of Epidemics . -. - (-), p1-9.

9. Tiensin, Thanawat . (2011). Epidemiology and Control of Avian Influenza H5N1 Virus in Thailand . PhD thesis, Faculty of Veterinary Medicine. - (-), p13-101.

10. World Health Organisation. (2012). Cumulative number of confirmed human cases for avian influenza A(H5N1) reported to WHO, 2003-2012. Available: http://www.who.int/influenza/human_animal_interface/EN_GIP_20121217CumulativeN umberH5N1cases.pdf. Last accessed 4th Jan 2013.